The Big Book of
WOULD YOU RATHER
Questions for Kids

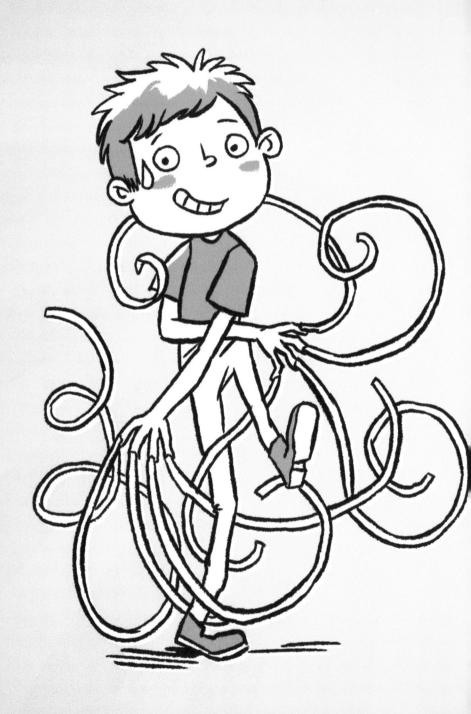

The Big Book of
Would You Rather
Questions for Kids

Over 350 Smart and Silly Scenarios

KEVIN KURTZ

ROCKRIDGE
PRESS

For general information on our other products and services or to obtain technical support, please contact our Customer Care Department within the United States at (866) 744-2665, or outside the United States at (510) 253-0500.

Rockridge Press publishes its books in a variety of electronic and print formats. Some content that appears in print may not be available in electronic books, and vice versa.

TRADEMARKS: Rockridge Press and the Rockridge Press logo are trademarks or registered trademarks of Callisto Media Inc. and/or its affiliates, in the United States and other countries, and may not be used without written permission. All other trademarks are the property of their respective owners. Rockridge Press is not associated with any product or vendor mentioned in this book.

Interior and Cover Designer: John Calmeyer
Art Producer: Hannah Dickerson
Editor: Barbara Isenberg
Production Editor: Jenna Dutton
Production Manager: Martin Worthington

Illustrations © 2021 Collaborate Agency
Decorative patterns used under license from iStock.com and Shutterstock.com
Author photo courtesy of Linda Saxton

Paperback ISBN: 978-1-63807-402-1
    eBook ISBN: 978-1-63807-236-2
R0

To Sarah, Adam, and Noah.
Thanks so much for all
the love, support, and goofiness.

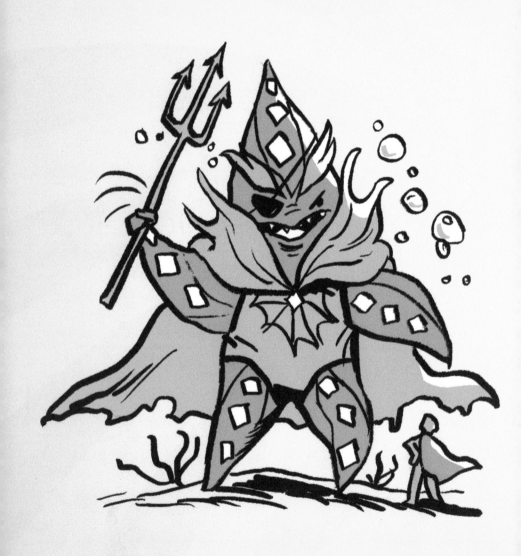

Contents

The Rules

Would you rather read the rules **OR** jump right into reading the questions?

Thank you for choosing to read the rules! Would You Rather is a fun game you can play with one other person, a bunch of other people, or alone. Would You Rather allows you to learn a lot about your friends, family, and even yourself. It's also fun because you get to imagine one another in some silly situations.

This book includes more than 350 Would You Rather questions for you and your friends and family to read and answer. The questions range from super silly (though hopefully not supercilious) to serious and thought-provoking.

This book is divided into 10 chapters. Each chapter contains a bunch of questions related to one topic, such as things that happen at school (School Scenes) or questions related to food (To Eat **OR** Not to Eat). The last chapter contains fill-in-the-blanks questions that allow you to come up with your own Would You Rather ideas. If at any point you come across a question that doesn't relate to you, feel free to skip it and move on to the next!

Would you rather play a game for fun **OR** play a game to win?

For either choice, Would You Rather is the game for you! If you're playing for fun, have someone read a question and then have everyone listening take turns answering it. Then enjoy the interesting, funny, and revealing conversations that begin! You can also read the book to have fun answering the questions by yourself.

If you are playing to win, here are the rules to follow:

1. Have all players get in a circle. Make sure each player has two small pieces of paper. One piece of paper should have "First Choice" written on it. The other piece of paper should have "Second Choice" written on it.

2. Choose someone to go first. After that, take turns going in clockwise order around the circle.

3. The first person to go will open the book to a random page and read a question. The person who goes next reads the next question and so on, until you have read all the questions on both pages. Then the next person in the circle will turn to another random page and start reading those questions.

4. After each question is read, the person whose turn it is to answer puts one of the pieces of paper in their right hand, hiding it from everyone else. If they are choosing the option before the **OR**, then they put their "First Choice" paper in their hand. If they are choosing the option after the **OR**, then they put the "Second Choice" paper in their hand.

5. Everyone else guesses whether the person who answered the question is more likely to pick the "First Choice" or the "Second Choice." Each of them puts the paper that matches their guess in their right hand.

6. When everyone has voted, all players reveal the paper in their right hand. Everyone whose answer matches that of the person answering the question gets a point. The players who guess wrong and the player whose turn it is do not get a point.

7. Keep score on another piece of paper. The first person to get 10 points is the winner. If there is a tie, keep playing until someone breaks the tie. Now, would you rather read even more rules **OR** start reading the questions? Hopefully, you chose "start reading the questions," because we're out of rules. Well, except one more.

8. Have fun!

1

DAILY DILEMMAS

WOULD YOU RATHER . . .

have to choose a different outfit
to wear for every day of the year
OR
wear the same outfit every day?

~~~~~~~~~~

brush your teeth by putting toothpaste on your finger
OR
squeezing the toothpaste directly into your mouth and
then using your tongue as the brush?

~~~~~~~~~~

leave the house barefoot
OR
wear tap shoes all day?

~~~~~~~~~~

wear a T-shirt that says,
"Here Comes Trouble"
OR
"My Grandma Went to Florida and
All I Got Was This Lousy T-Shirt"?

~~~~~~~~~~

be woken up by having a marching band
play outside your room
OR
a spring-loaded bed fling you into a pool?

WOULD YOU RATHER . . .

have 50 different pairs of
underwear to choose from
OR
50 different pairs of socks?

your home had a microwave but not a dishwasher
OR
a dishwasher but not a microwave?

have to make your bed every day
OR
get rid of the bed and sleep on the floor?

your house always smelled like coffee
OR
your parents always smelled like coffee?

have only one hour of screen time a day
OR
no screen time, but four hours a day
to do whatever else you feel like?

WOULD YOU RATHER . . .

go shopping for clothes
OR
fire extinguishers?

have two bathrooms in your home
OR
two TVs?

have a refrigerator in your room
OR
a bigger bed?

wear hand-me-down clothes
OR
handmade clothes?

have your allowance paid in diamonds
OR
gift cards?

get clean by taking a bath
OR
running through a car wash?

WOULD YOU RATHER . . .

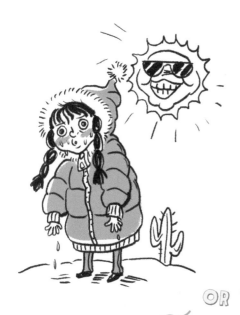

wear a winter coat on a hot summer day

OR

shorts and a T-shirt on a cold winter day?

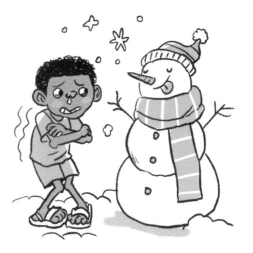

WOULD YOU RATHER . . .

post videos online of yourself dancing
OR
you and your family shopping
for slime ingredients?

your parents do all the cooking and cleaning
for meals, even though it's food you don't like,
OR
you always have your favorite dishes for meals,
but you do all the cooking and cleaning up?

live in a huge house with a loud
highway right behind it
OR
a small house with a forest right behind it?

live like your parents did when they were kids
OR
your grandparents did when they were kids?

that all the bandages in your house
have pictures of vultures on them
OR
pictures of vacuum cleaners?

Would you rather . . .

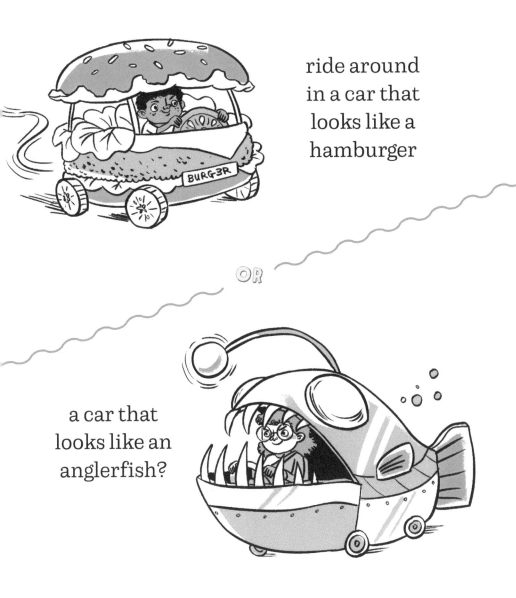

ride around
in a car that
looks like a
hamburger

OR

a car that
looks like an
anglerfish?

WOULD YOU RATHER . . .

have a remote control to raise and lower the
volume of all the devices in your house

OR

all the people in your house?

have posters hanging up in your
room of famous pirates

OR

gold-medal-winning bobsledders?

that your parents had something fun
planned for you to do every day

OR

that some days they had nothing planned for
you and you could do what you want?

read only books that list world record holders

OR

read only books in which one of
the characters is a raccoon?

WOULD YOU RATHER . . .

have to mow the lawn around
your home every week

~~~~~~~ OR ~~~~~~~

not have anyone mow the lawn and a pack
of wolves moves into your yard?

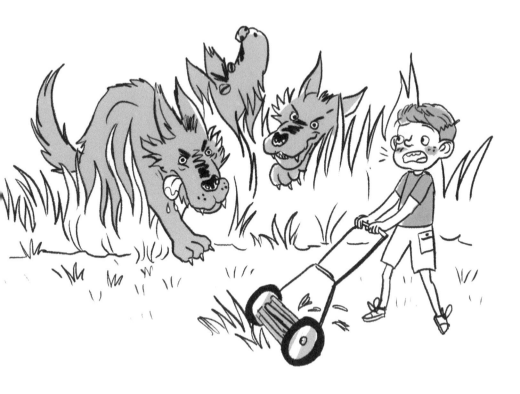

WOULD YOU RATHER . . .

have a night-light to make walking around
the house in the middle of the night less scary
OR
have a mastery of martial arts to make walking
around the house in the middle of the night less scary?

~~~~~~~

your shampoo smelled like hot dogs
OR
diesel fumes?

~~~~~~~

have neighbors who are too loud
OR
who keep telling you to stop being loud?

~~~~~~~

have a five-dollar bill in your bank
OR
550 pennies?

~~~~~~~

have your own treehouse
OR
your own secret room with a
hidden door in your home?

WOULD YOU RATHER . . .

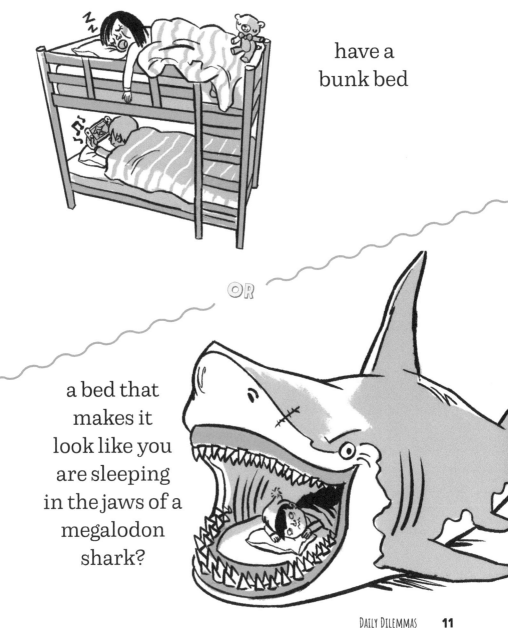

have a
bunk bed

OR

a bed that
makes it
look like you
are sleeping
in the jaws of a
megalodon
shark?

Would you rather . . .

your home had hard floors you
could slide on in socks

OR

soft carpets you could lie down on?

always be the one who chooses the
music your family listens to

OR

the TV shows your family watches?

have your bedroom next to the bedrooms
of everyone else in your home

OR

as far from all the other bedrooms as possible?

take a nap every day

OR

never take a nap ever again?

WOULD YOU RATHER . . .

always be able to sit in the
front seat of a car

~~~~~ OR ~~~~~

sit on a throne on a parade float
that is being pulled by the car?

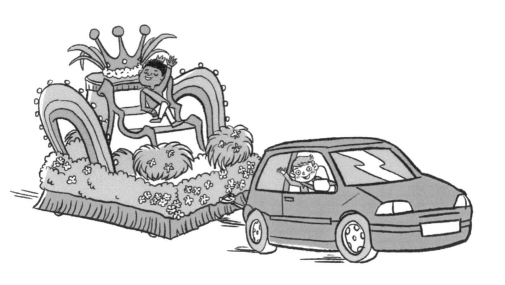

2

ALL ABOUT YOU

WOULD YOU RATHER . . .

your hiccups made the normal "hic" sound
OR
that every hiccup sounds like the blast of an airhorn?

be taller than everyone else in your house
OR
louder?

your age was the same number as your weight
OR
that your age was the same number as your shoe size?

be the fastest talker at your school
OR
the fastest eater?

have green hair
OR
purple eyes?

WOULD YOU RATHER . . .

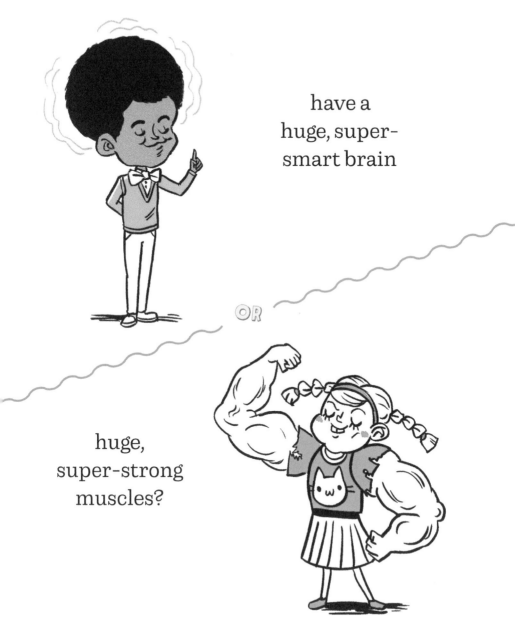

have a
huge, super-
smart brain

OR

huge,
super-strong
muscles?

WOULD YOU RATHER . . .

have a photographic memory (meaning
you literally remember everything)
OR
a photogenic face (meaning your face
always looks good in photographs)?

~~~~~~~~~~~~~~~~~~~~~~~~~~~~

smell like perfume/cologne all the time
OR
nothing?

~~~~~~~~~~~~~~~~~~~~~~~~~~~~

have huge arm muscles
OR
huge leg muscles?

~~~~~~~~~~~~~~~~~~~~~~~~~~~~

only breathe through your nose
OR
your mouth?

~~~~~~~~~~~~~~~~~~~~~~~~~~~~

have a great sense of rhythm,
so you can dance and play music,
OR
a great sense of balance, so you can walk
across balance beams and ride a bike without
having your hands on the handlebars?

Would you rather . . .

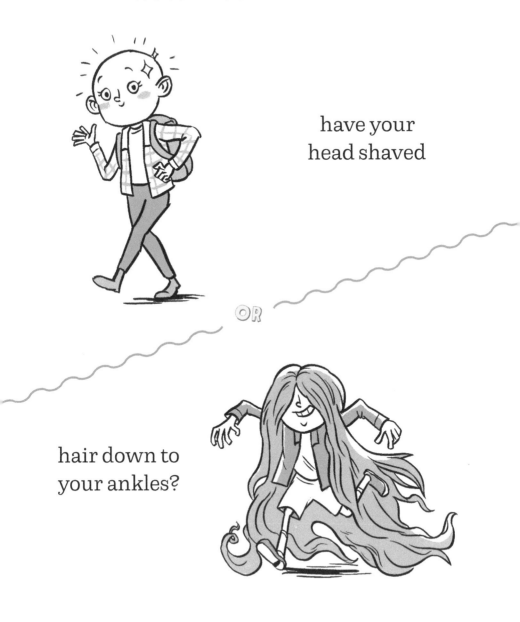

have your
head shaved

OR

hair down to
your ankles?

WOULD YOU RATHER . . .

have shiny knees
OR
shiny elbows?

always be clean
OR
always be funny?

have a stomachache
OR
a headache?

get a charley horse while running
OR
a side stitch?

be able to throw a baseball with pinpoint accuracy
OR
a snowball?

WOULD YOU RATHER . . .

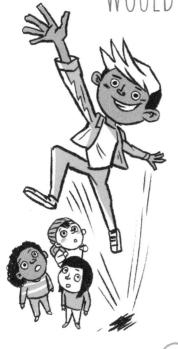

jump high
enough to touch
the ceiling

OR

bend backward
low enough
to win every
limbo contest?

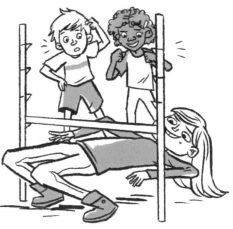

WOULD YOU RATHER . . .

have thick hair and no eyebrows
OR
thick eyebrows and no hair?

never sweat
OR
never drool?

spend eight hours a day sleeping
and two hours a day eating
OR
four hours a day sleeping and six hours a day eating?

lose the ability to taste sour stuff
OR
Brussels sprouts?

never feel nervous
OR
never feel sad?

WOULD YOU RATHER . . .

feel the need to dance every
time you hear music

~~~~~~~~ OR ~~~~~~~~

sing every time
you hear music?

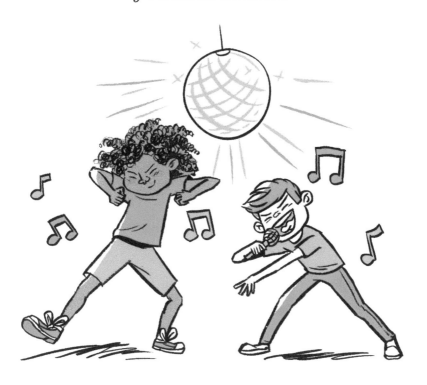

WOULD YOU RATHER . . .

have such powerful hearing that you can
hear people whispering in another room

OR

ears with an on/off button so sometimes
you don't have to hear anything?

be the best at drawing at school

OR

at rapping?

never have to cut your hair

OR

your fingernails?

be able to sing a high note that could break glass

OR

have a voice so deep you can use it to
warn ships in foggy weather?

your fingers couldn't be burned
by touching something hot

OR

your mouth couldn't be burned by
tasting something hot?

WOULD YOU RATHER . . .

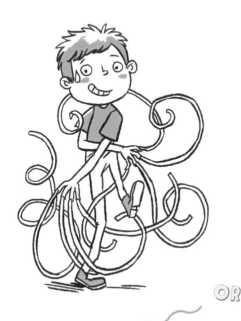

hold the world record for having the longest fingernails

OR

for being able to stick the most billiard balls into your mouth?

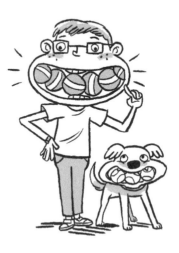

Would you rather . . .

be able to sneeze without making a sound

OR

without anything actually
coming out of your nose or mouth?

be able to run really fast only
when you're racing other kids

OR

only when you're being chased by bees?

sleepwalk and just wander around

OR

do your homework while you sleepwalk?

your laugh always make everyone else laugh

OR

the look on your face always
make everyone else laugh?

wear glasses

OR

contact lenses?

WOULD YOU RATHER . . .

have all sharp teeth, so it is easier for you to eat meat,
OR
all hard, flat teeth, so it easier to eat
crunchy food like peanuts and apples?

snore all night, every night
OR
occasionally wake up screaming
at 3:00 in the morning?

have the bottoms of your bare feet
be so tough that you can walk on rocks
without it bothering you
OR
be soft enough that it feels really
good when they are tickled?

be great at snapping your fingers
OR
whistling?

3

SCHOOL SCENES

WOULD YOU RATHER . . .

your school had a four-square team you could join

OR

a table-tennis team?

your school was on top of the
world's tallest skyscraper

OR

hidden in a secret underground tunnel?

your school mascot was a unicorn

OR

a chipmunk?

wear 10-year-old sneakers to school

OR

bring a 10-year-old phone to school?

trade places with the principal for a day

OR

one of the custodians?

WOULD YOU RATHER . . .

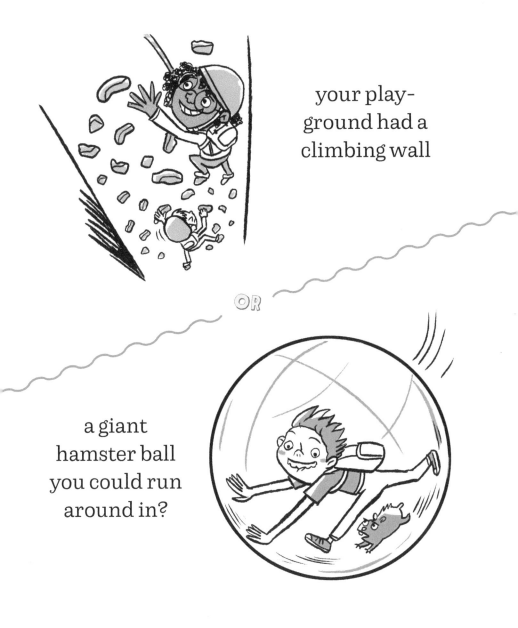

your play-
ground had a
climbing wall

OR

a giant
hamster ball
you could run
around in?

WOULD YOU RATHER . . .

keep all your stuff in a locker on the other
side of the school from your classes
OR
carry all your stuff with you wherever you go?

your teacher was too nice
OR
too mean?

have gym class outside
OR
math class?

have a children's author visit your school
OR
a group of performers who do yo-yo tricks?

have a fire drill interrupt classes
on every day of the school year
OR
only on days when the weather outside is perfect?

WOULD YOU RATHER . . .

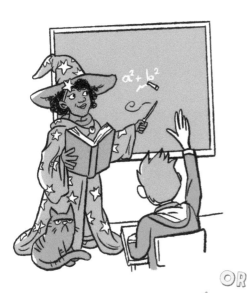

go to a school
where all
the teachers
are wizards

OR

go to a school
where all
the teachers
are superheroes?

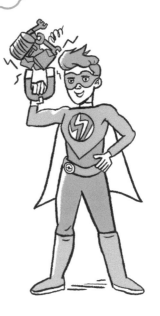

WOULD YOU RATHER . . .

play a tooth in a school play
OR
a carrot?

the school had to call your parents
because you threw up
OR
because your pants ripped in half?

your lunch period was at 9:30 in the morning
OR
at 2:00 in the afternoon?

that loud music is played and bright lights
flash to announce your arrival to a classroom
OR
that you come in through a secret door
in the back so that no one notices you?

your school had its own swimming pool
OR
bowling alley?

WOULD YOU RATHER . . .

Have drones fly you
to school every day

~~~~~~~~~~ OR ~~~~~~~~~~

be pulled to school
by sled dogs?

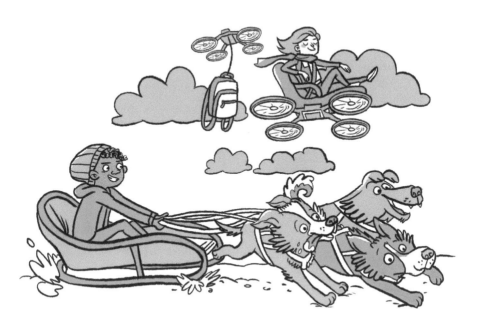

WOULD YOU RATHER . . .

you could bring pets with you to school

OR

parents?

~~~~~~~~~~~~~~~~~~~~~~~~

that the school band, chorus, and teachers perform and
sing "Happy Birthday" to you on your birthday

OR

someone just gives you a cupcake?

~~~~~~~~~~~~~~~~~~~~~~~~

the students had to make all the food in the cafeteria

OR

clean all the classrooms, hallways, and bathrooms?

~~~~~~~~~~~~~~~~~~~~~~~~

your teacher always called everyone
in the classroom "friends"

OR

"children"?

~~~~~~~~~~~~~~~~~~~~~~~~

eat in the school cafeteria for a week

OR

have your parents pack you a healthy
lunch every day that week?

WOULD YOU RATHER . . .

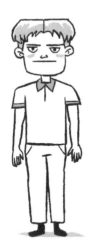

your school had
a uniform policy
where everyone has
to wear tan bottoms
with white tops

OR

a uniform
policy where
everyone has
to wear 1970s
disco outfits?

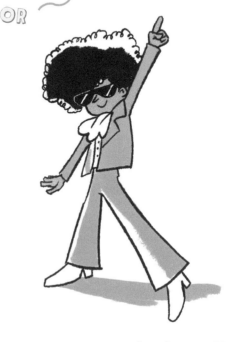

WOULD YOU RATHER . . .

stay at school an extra hour each day
and never have homework
OR
keep the same school schedule and still have homework?

your school was four stories high
OR
one story high but half a mile long?

your school library had a bunch of
books signed by famous authors
OR
thousands of graphic novels to choose from?

your parents could go online every day to check
your grades
OR
not know your grades until your report card came out?

see your teacher in a store
OR
your principal?

Would you rather . . .

baby chicks escape
from science class

~~~~~~~~~ OR ~~~~~~~~~

iguanas escape
from science class?

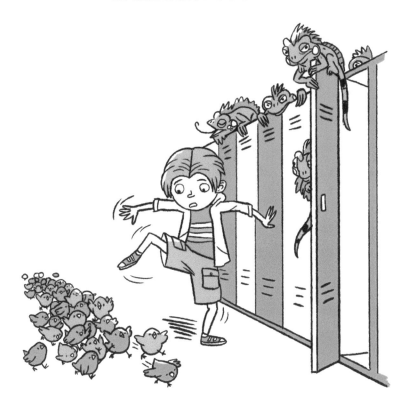

WOULD YOU RATHER . . .

not get any snow or bad-weather days off but
instead get guaranteed days off like National
Bean Day and Talk Like a Pirate Day

OR

keep the chance of getting occasional snow or
bad-weather days off with no additional holidays?

ride on a school bus for two hours straight

OR

write on a marker board "I will not make fun
of school buses" 200 times in a row?

get accidentally hit in the head
during gym class by a softball

OR

a plastic hockey stick?

be able to hang out on the
school's roof for a day

OR

in the teacher's lounge?

Would you rather . . .

be most famous in your school for
being able to draw anime characters

OR

burp the alphabet?

~~~~~~~~

sit in the nurse's office for half an hour by yourself
on a vinyl cushion while wearing shorts

OR

not tell anyone you don't feel well?

~~~~~~~~

go on a field trip to an aquarium

OR

a factory that makes cookies?

~~~~~~~~

one of your parents was your regular
teacher who teaches you every school day

OR

your art teacher who you see once a week?

~~~~~~~~

walk eight blocks to school

OR

ride a subway there?

4

AROUND
THE WORLD

Would you rather . . .

sit on a plane next to a crying baby

OR

a sleeping guy who keeps
snoring the entire trip?

visit a museum about bananas

OR

mustard?

go the ancient Colosseum in Rome, Italy

OR

a football stadium named after the Colosseum?

go to an amusement park with a bunch
of cartoon characters that were popular
when your grandparents were kids

OR

characters no one has ever heard of?

stay in a hotel that has an indoor swimming pool

OR

Wi-Fi in your room?

WOULD YOU RATHER . . .

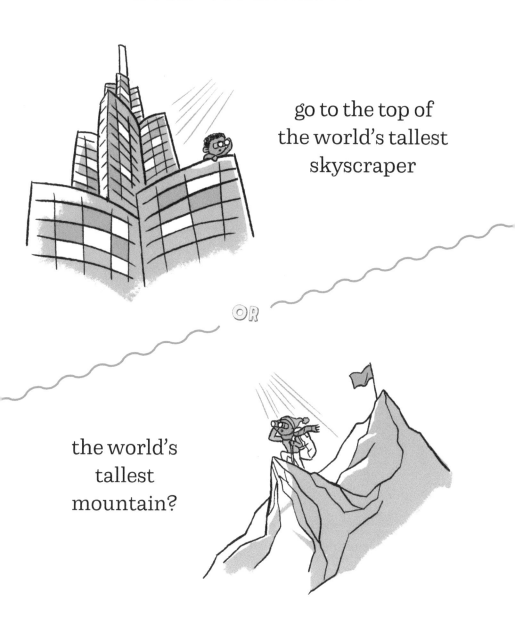

go to the top of
the world's tallest
skyscraper

OR

the world's
tallest
mountain?

WOULD YOU RATHER . . .

ride in a car for 1,000 miles and
have only one movie to watch

OR

one video game to play?

go to a beach where it is too cold to swim, but you can
explore tide pools and see sea lions and other animals

OR

where it is warm enough to swim, but you are
surrounded by hundreds of people and the
only animals around are seagulls?

go on a vacation with your family where
you all wear matching custom-made
T-shirts with your family's name on it

OR

where you all purchase and wear T-shirts that
say the name of the place you are visiting?

visit another country

OR

an amusement park where part of
it is made to look like that other country?

WOULD YOU RATHER . . .

ride a mule down to the bottom of the Grand Canyon
OR
a camel around the Egyptian pyramids?

go to a place where you can swim with dolphins
OR
penguins?

go to another country and try as many
of the local foods as you can
OR
go to another country and eat only
in American chain restaurants?

be on a cruise ship surrounded by icebergs
OR
sharks?

go on vacation with someone who
mainly wants to bungee-jump
OR
someone who only wants
to nap on the beach?

WOULD YOU RATHER . . .

go to a restaurant owned by a famous chef

OR

go see your favorite actor's handprints
imprinted in a sidewalk?

---

stay in a place that is in walking distance to a beach

OR

an ice-cream stand?

---

see a geyser erupt

OR

your family members erupt out of
a waterslide tube at a water park?

---

go on safari and see the scariest land
predators in their natural habitats

OR

go scuba diving and see the scariest ocean
predators in their natural habitats?

---

go somewhere really hot in the summer

OR

really cold in the winter?

WOULD YOU RATHER . . .

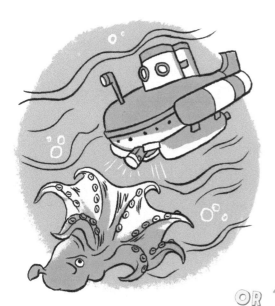

ride in a submersible that takes you to the deepest place in the ocean

OR

on a space tourism flight that takes you into orbit around Earth?

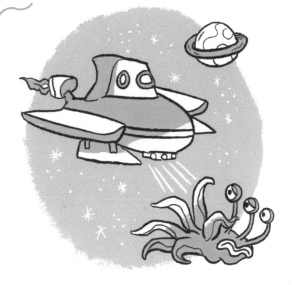

WOULD YOU RATHER . . .

go to an amusement park that has amazing
rides, but you spend 12 of your 14 hours
there waiting in line to get on them

OR

an amusement park where you
don't have to wait in line at all,
but the rides are kind of boring?

~~~~~~~~~~~

go see the world's biggest ball of twine

OR

biggest ball of rubber bands?

~~~~~~~~~~~

go on vacation to another country
for a week and try to see as many different
places across that country as you can

OR

spend all week exploring just one
small part of that country?

~~~~~~~~~~~

go on a vacation where your
main goal is to get a tan

OR

go shopping?

WOULD YOU RATHER . . .

go on a vacation to a boring place
in the middle of nowhere

OR

on a cruise ship through
the Bermuda Triangle?

visit a real medieval castle in Europe

OR

go to a fair where everyone is dressed
and acting like they live in a European medieval
castle, except you're nowhere near Europe?

plan your family vacation for weeks in advance

OR

just go somewhere and wing it?

come back from vacation and tell your friends
some historic facts about the places you visited

OR

share how toilets work in different countries?

WOULD YOU RATHER . . .

visit Ding Dong, Texas,

OR

Idiotville, Oregon?

go on vacation to a place that thousands
of other tourists are also visiting

OR

a place that you have all to yourself?

fly across an ocean

OR

take a cruise across it?

go to a museum where you can see the
most famous painting in the world

OR

the first spaceship that landed
people on the moon?

WOULD YOU RATHER . . .

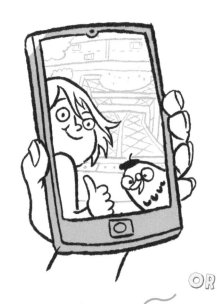

take a selfie from
the top of the
Eiffel Tower

OR

the Great
Wall of China?

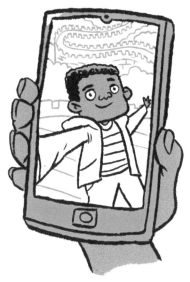

WOULD YOU RATHER . . .

visit a national park where you can
get up close to herds of bison

OR

visit a museum where you can get
up close to Abraham Lincoln's pants?

vacation in a place that has
gift shops everywhere

OR

no gift shops at all?

ski in an indoor ski resort in Dubai

OR

ski on the most dangerous
slopes in the Alps?

hike near a grizzly bear

OR

hike near a lava flow on an active volcano?

WOULD YOU RATHER . . .

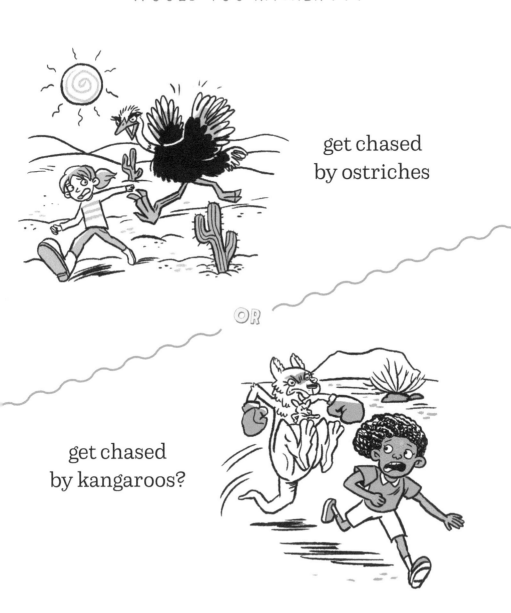

get chased
by ostriches

OR

get chased
by kangaroos?

5

To Eat Or Not to Eat

WOULD YOU RATHER . . .

have to eat meat loaf for breakfast
OR
mashed potatoes?

eat in a restaurant where the staff tries
to throw shrimp in your mouth
OR
broccoli?

sprinkle sugar on everything you eat
OR
salt?

eat deep-fried cheesecake
OR
deep-fried jellybeans?

eat strawberries you picked yourself
OR
fish you caught yourself?

Would you rather . . .

know how to make mac and cheese
OR
pancakes?

eat cereal for three meals a day
OR
pizza?

that every week your family
has Sushi Sunday
OR
Three-Bean-Salad Thursday?

eat a waffle shaped like a butterfly
OR
the state of Texas?

eat a leftover burrito
OR
leftover French fries?

WOULD YOU RATHER . . .

eat in a restaurant where the server
asks to grind pepper on your salad
OR
asks, "Do you want fries with that?"

eat only bananas for a week
OR
cheese sticks?

try garlic-flavored ice cream
OR
sweet corn–flavored?

never drink milk again
OR
never eat bread again?

eat a pizza with pineapple on it
OR
lettuce?

WOULD YOU RATHER . . .

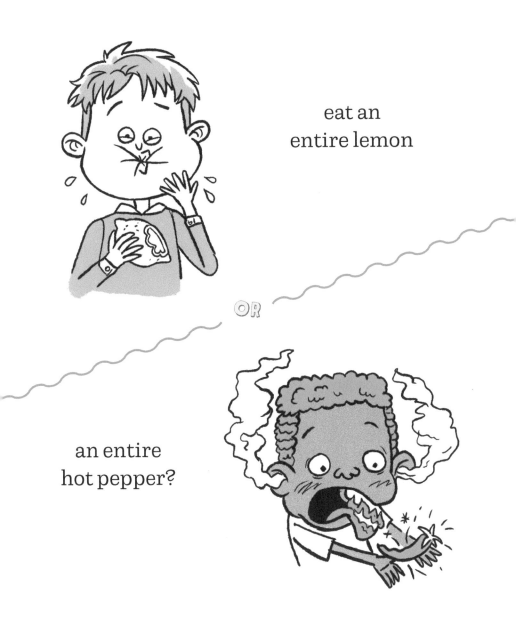

eat an
entire lemon

OR

an entire
hot pepper?

WOULD YOU RATHER . . .

drink a really thick milkshake through a straw
OR
eat a thin milkshake with a spoon?

eat a cheeseburger without the cheese
OR
without the burger?

every sandwich you eat from now
on had mayonnaise on it
OR
peanut butter?

go trick-or-treating to get a bag
full of random candy
OR
just have someone buy you a large
bag of your favorite candy?

eat pickled fish
OR
pickled beets?

Would you rather . . .

eat soup with your hands

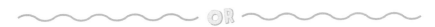

OR

steak with a spoon?

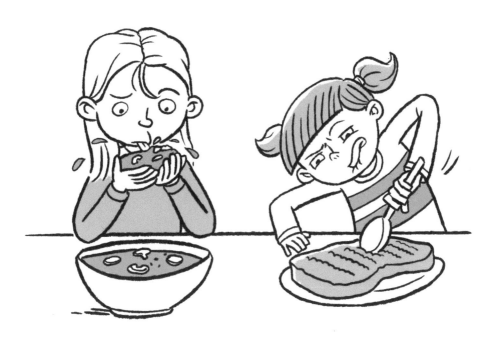

WOULD YOU RATHER . . .

be lost in the woods and have to eat tree bark

OR

lily pads?

~~~~~~~~~~

eat your favorite food every day

OR

only have it on special occasions?

~~~~~~~~~~

eat only food that is cooked in a microwave

OR

on a grill?

~~~~~~~~~~

eat chocolate-covered ants

OR

caramelized onions?

~~~~~~~~~~

have a secret stash of candy in your house

OR

a secret stash of chicken tenders?

WOULD YOU RATHER . . .

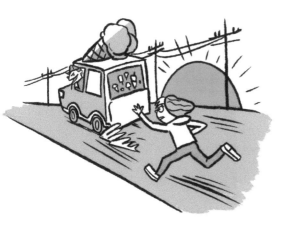

chase an
ice-cream truck
to buy some
ice cream

OR

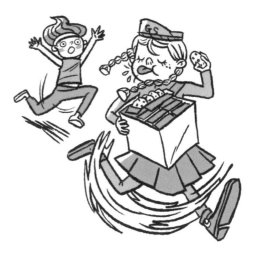

chase a
Girl Scout
to buy
some cookies?

WOULD YOU RATHER . . .

eat three filling meals a day
OR
nine mini-meals?

have a salad bar in your house
OR
a seafood buffet?

eat until you feel sick at holiday dinners
OR
eat only the salad?

eat something super-spicy hot
OR
get brain freeze?

see that food in the fridge went bad
OR
smell that it went bad?

WOULD YOU RATHER . . .

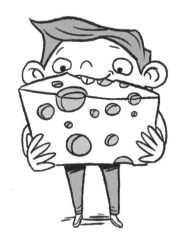

eat a block of
cheese bigger than
your head

OR

a watermelon
bigger than
your head?

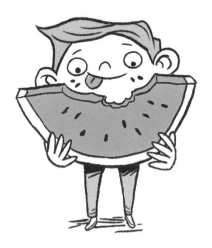

WOULD YOU RATHER . . .

eat high-fructose corn syrup
OR
monosodium glutamate?
(check the ingredients list on your
snack food to help you decide)

~~~~~~~~~~~~~~~

eat cold chili
OR
warm ice cream?

~~~~~~~~~~~~~~~

eat dog food
OR
cat food?

~~~~~~~~~~~~~~~

eat a hamburger made out of plants
OR
made out of meat that was grown in a laboratory?

~~~~~~~~~~~~~~~

eat food that turns your tongue yellow
OR
green?

6

Sports and Hobbies

WOULD YOU RATHER . . .

listen to someone play a trombone
for three hours straight
OR
the bongos for three hours straight?

get a book that's guaranteed to be your
favorite of all time when you read it
OR
not read any books for three months?

play many different sports as a kid
OR
play only one sport your entire childhood,
but be really good at it?

watch a movie in a movie theater
OR
on a phone?

WOULD YOU RATHER . . .

play catch with a friend in the street

OR

while both of you are standing on the
roofs of two different buildings?

have your own horse to ride

OR

your own hang glider?

have your room decorated to show
who your favorite sports team is

OR

what your favorite movie is?

have a black belt in martial arts

OR

a trophy for Most Valuable Player for a sports team?

WOULD YOU RATHER . . .

get a building block set and always follow
the instructions to make things

OR

come up with your own ideas of what to make?

listen only to music that is popular right now

OR

sometimes listen to music that no one
else at your school knows about?

go on a singing competition show

OR

a baking competition show?

learn how to knit your own socks

OR

sculpt your own hot-cocoa mug?

listen to your favorite band play a song live

OR

have your bowling ball knock down 10 pins at once?

WOULD YOU RATHER . . .

that Olympic divers got more points for making the smallest splash

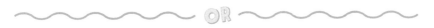 OR

for making the biggest splash?

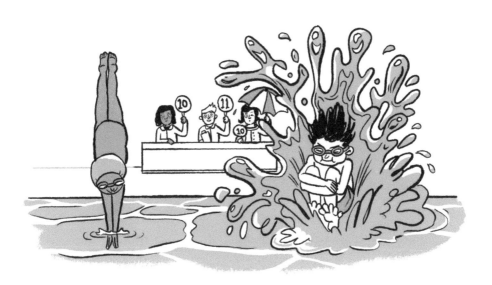

WOULD YOU RATHER . . .

start a garden so you could grow cucumbers
OR
sunflowers?

play your favorite sport on a team where you
play only in practices and never in games
OR
not play the sport at all?

play hide and seek inside an
empty school building
OR
in a cornfield?

make yourself run faster in a race
by thinking about winning
OR
thinking about being chased by zombies?

your gamer name was "SteelCockroach"
OR
"Giblets5000"?

WOULD YOU RATHER . . .

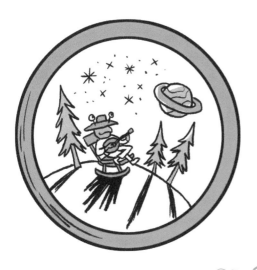

have a powerful telescope that allows you to see other planets

OR

a powerful microscope that allows you to see what microbes are living on your skin?

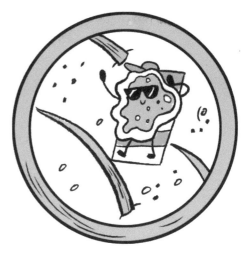

WOULD YOU RATHER . . .

play basketball in the school gym
OR
with a rim low enough
that everyone can slam dunk?

live in a place where it is cold enough that you
can ski, sled, and skate in the winter
OR
where "winter sports" just means
you dress a little warmer when you
play sports outside because it is not cold
enough for there to be snow and ice there?

be known for having the world's largest
collection of tissue boxes
OR
banana stickers?

go fishing and catch a high-heeled shoe
OR
a Bundt cake pan?

Would you rather . . .

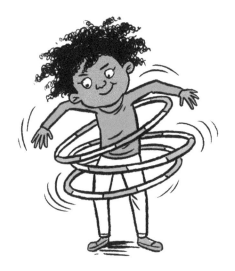

be able to
hula hoop for
10 minutes

OR

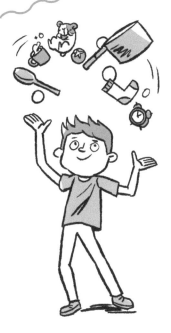

juggle for
10 minutes?

WOULD YOU RATHER . . .

learn to play an instrument so
you can be a solo performer
OR
play in a band?

watch a black-and-white movie
OR
a movie with subtitles?

play volleyball with a ball
OR
a rubber chicken?

play basketball in a pool
OR
play Marco Polo on a basketball court?

body surf until you throw up
OR
jump on a trampoline until you throw up?

WOULD YOU RATHER . . .

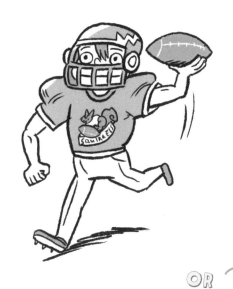

be the quarterback of the football team

OR

the team's costumed mascot?

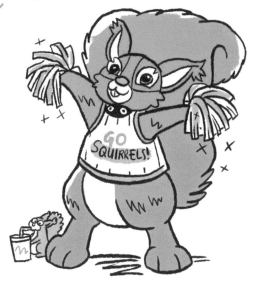

Would you rather . . .

make your own songs
OR
your own comics?

use a melon for a soccer ball
OR
a zucchini for a baseball bat?

have one solo win on a multiplayer video game
OR
four wins as part of a squad?

be the best kickball player in your county
OR
the best badminton player?

Would you rather . . .

binge-watch an entire season of
a TV show in one weekend

OR

wait a week to watch each new episode?

have a baseball bat engineered to hit the ball farther

OR

a baseball glove engineered to be better at not
dropping balls?

run for 15 minutes in your neighborhood

OR

on a treadmill?

play "Would You Rather" with your family

OR

read a book of "Would You Rather"
questions by yourself?

7

ANIMALS AND
OTHER CREATURES

WOULD YOU RATHER . . .

be a yellow-bellied sapsucker
OR
a blue-footed booby?

have a bunch of bees living in your yard
OR
a bunch of garter snakes?

be able to run as fast as a cheetah
OR
swim as fast as a tuna?

be an animal that eats grass
OR
an animal that eats squirrels?

be an animal that spends most of its
life in a group, like wildebeests,
OR
alone, like a woodchuck?

WOULD YOU RATHER . . .

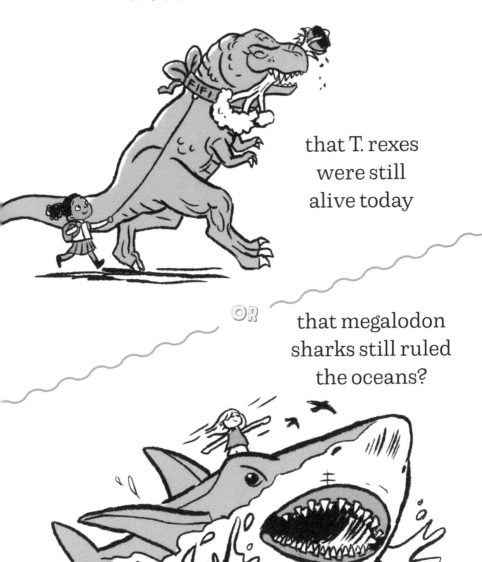

that T. rexes were still alive today

OR

that megalodon sharks still ruled the oceans?

WOULD YOU RATHER . . .

have a llama as a pet
OR
a colony of naked mole rats?

~~~~~~~~~~

have a bird feeder outside your window
OR
a bear feeder?

~~~~~~~~~~

be a baby in a kangaroo pouch
OR
a baby in a seahorse pouch?

~~~~~~~~~~

live in a house infested with spiders
OR
cockroaches?

~~~~~~~~~~

live the life of a dog
OR
a cat?

Would you rather . . .

have a watchdog protecting the outside of your home
OR
a watchskunk?

drink milk from an anteater
OR
a moose?

have a ranch full of unicorns
OR
an aquarium full of mermaids?

find out the Loch Ness Monster is a
plesiosaur that somehow escaped extinction
OR
find out it's a prank that has been pulled
on the world by a Scottish family for decades?

WOULD YOU RATHER . . .

be a bird that gets all its food from
a backyard bird feeder

OR

be a bird that must find all its food in a forest?

live in an elaborate nest in a tree, like a hornet,

OR

in elaborate underground tunnels, like an ant?

be a flying squirrel

OR

a flying fish?

be an animal that flies thousands of miles
to go south every winter, like a goose,

OR

an animal that basically sleeps all winter, like a bear?

have to take care of an elephant

OR

a humpback whale?

Would you rather . . .

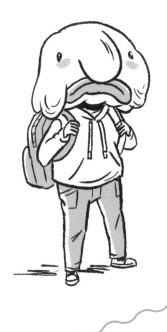

go through life
looking like a
blobfish out
of water

OR

turn into a
warthog?

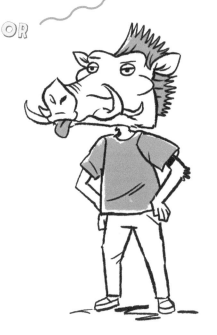

Would you rather . . .

be able to make sounds like a mockingbird

OR

a howler monkey?

protect yourself from bullies by
playing dead like a possum

OR

inflating your body like a blowfish?

be stuck in a cage for an hour with a boa constrictor

OR

an aggressive chicken?

bang your head against a tree all day, like a woodpecker,

OR

push around large balls of poop
all day, like a dung beetle?

WOULD YOU RATHER . . .

that rabbits be the
dominant animals on Earth

OR

that frogs reign supreme?

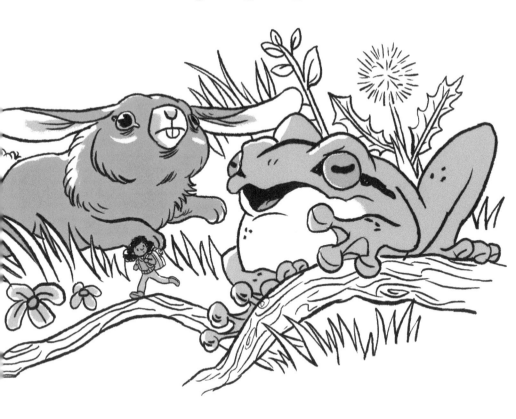

WOULD YOU RATHER . . .

see Bigfoot in the woods
OR
only in blurry photos
in books and on websites?

~~~~~~~~

ride a giraffe
OR
an ostrich?

~~~~~~~~

wear a T-shirt that shows a wolf howling at the moon
OR
a dolphin jumping out of the water
in front of a rainbow?

~~~~~~~~

go to a beach that has hundreds of sharks in the water
OR
hundreds of jellyfish?

WOULD YOU RATHER . . .

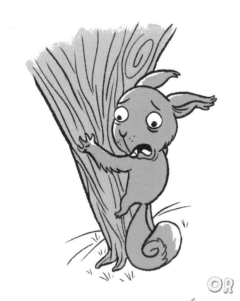

be a squirrel
that is afraid
of heights

OR

an ant that is
afraid of being
in crowds?

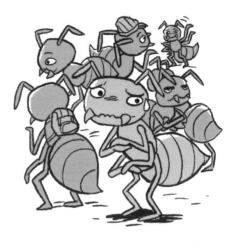

Would you rather . . .

be a snail and have your own shell

OR

a hermit crab that has to shell-hop
and find new shells your entire life?

~~~~~~~~~~~~~~~~

sleep for more than 20 hours a day like a koala

OR

sleep just a few hours a day, but your
eyes are always open, like a fish?

~~~~~~~~~~~~~~~~

be a wizard who has an owl as
your magical animal friend

OR

a raccoon?

~~~~~~~~~~~~~~~~

watch a webcam on a sea turtle's back

OR

a zebra's?

Would you rather . . .

be a dolphin using echolocation to find fish
OR
a bat using echolocation to find bugs?

not be able to go anywhere, like an oyster,
OR
not have a brain, like a jellyfish?

be a warm-blooded animal that can live anywhere
OR
a cold-blooded animal that can
only live in hot, sunny places?

be the world's tallest giraffe
OR
the world's shortest dachshund?

Superpowers
and Skills

WOULD YOU RATHER . . .

be Beaverperson, a superhero whose
superpowers are like the abilities of a beaver,

OR

Duckperson, a superhero whose superpowers
are like the abilities of a duck?

~~~~~~~~~~

have eyes that can see faraway things, like a telescope,

OR

tiny things, like a microscope?

~~~~~~~~~~

be able to make it rain whenever you want

OR

snow?

~~~~~~~~~~

be able to talk to and understand animals

OR

microbes?

~~~~~~~~~~

have metal claws that can shoot out of your hand

OR

metal forks, so you're always ready to eat?

WOULD YOU RATHER . . .

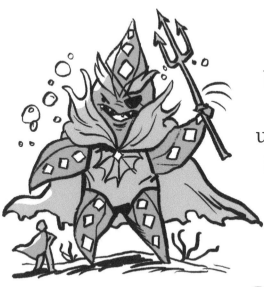

be a superhero who breathes underwater and fights crime in the ocean

OR

who can live without water and fights crime in the desert?

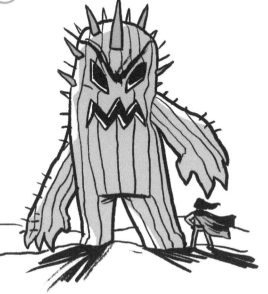

Would you rather . . .

be able to walk on your hands

OR

grab things with your feet?

~~~~~~~~~~~~~~~~~~~~~~~~~~~~~

be able to turn yourself invisible

OR

turn other things invisible?

~~~~~~~~~~~~~~~~~~~~~~~~~~~~~

have the strength to squeeze coal into diamonds

OR

the telepathic ability to turn
mean people into nice people?

~~~~~~~~~~~~~~~~~~~~~~~~~~~~~

get superpowers by being too close
to a nuclear bomb explosion

OR

bitten by a radioactive insect?

~~~~~~~~~~~~~~~~~~~~~~~~~~~~~

be able to stretch your body into any shape

OR

transform your body into any animal?

WOULD YOU RATHER . . .

get your superpowers from
a magic ring you keep losing

OR

a magic word you have
trouble pronouncing?

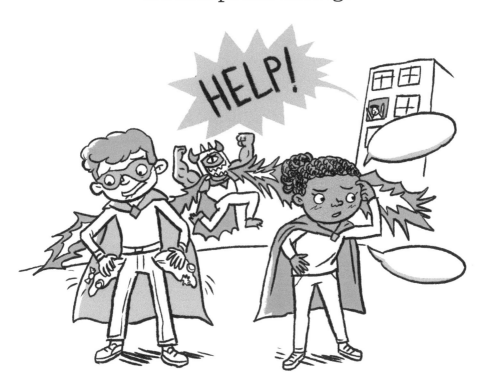

WOULD YOU RATHER . . .

have a magic tongue that makes everything taste good

OR

a magic nose that makes everything smell good?

be able to time travel but only go into the future

OR

the past?

have superpowers because you
were born on another planet

OR

not have superpowers, but be so incredibly
rich that you can get all the training and
technology you need to become a superhero?

be able to touch anyone and learn
all about their history

OR

gain their powers, even if it's
the power to be a dentist?

be able to shoot lasers out of your eyes

OR

your index fingers?

Would you rather . . .

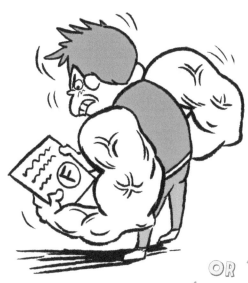

transform into an incredibly muscular superhero whenever you get angry

OR

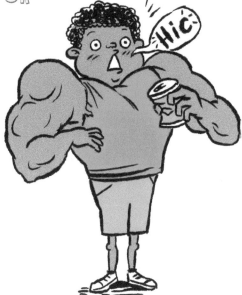

whenever you get the hiccups?

WOULD YOU RATHER . . .

have the magical ability to read other people's minds
OR
make everyone you talk to always
listen to what you say?

~~~~~~~~~~

fight crime as Doctor Odor, with
your ability to produce any smell,
OR
as Captain Cookie, with your ability to
make cookies appear out of nowhere?

~~~~~~~~~~

have the brain of a 10-year-old
in the body of a 30-year-old
OR
the brain of a 30-year-old in the
body of a 10-year-old?

~~~~~~~~~~

have the ability to speed time up
OR
make time stop?

~~~~~~~~~~

be able to make bees do whatever you want
OR
blue jays?

WOULD YOU RATHER . . .

always have an invisible force field in front of
you to prevent things from running into you

OR

above you to prevent things that drop
from the sky from falling on your head?

have the power to attract metals near you to your body

OR

any ice cream near you to your mouth?

be the Human Air Conditioner, who
can make anything around you cooler,

OR

the Human Furnace, who can make
anything around you warmer?

be able to start fires with the wave of your hand

OR

put out fires with a wave of your hand?

WOULD YOU RATHER . . .

have really long hair that can grab
things and pick them up

OR

a tail that can do the same thing?

have a sixth sense that tells you
when danger is nearby

OR

when free food is nearby?

be able to become 50 feet tall instantly,
except your clothes don't grow with you,
so you're a 50-foot-tall naked person

OR

shrink down to 1 inch and get lost in your clothes?

be half human and half fish

OR

half human and half bat?

be able to spin around until you make a tornado

OR

splash around in water until you make a tsunami?

WOULD YOU RATHER . . .

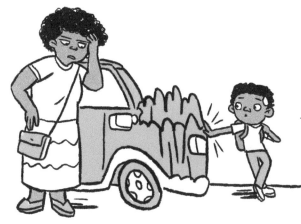

your body
was as hard
as steel

OR

as bouncy as a
rubber ball?

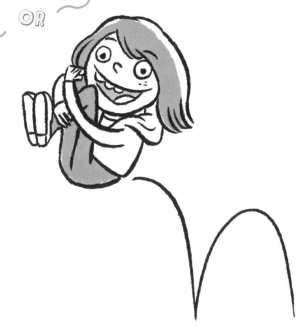

WOULD YOU RATHER . . .

be invulnerable to physical pain
OR
having your feelings hurt?

~~~~~~~~~

have two heads
OR
four arms?

~~~~~~~~~

be able to go into other people's dreams
OR
project your own dreams like a movie
so everyone can watch them?

~~~~~~~~~

be able to change your face to look like anyone else
OR
your voice to sound like anyone else?

~~~~~~~~~

be able to hypnotize people, but the only thing
you can make them do is act like chickens,
OR
the only thing you can make
them do is stop being mad?

WOULD YOU RATHER . . .

be able
to walk
up walls

OR

through
walls?

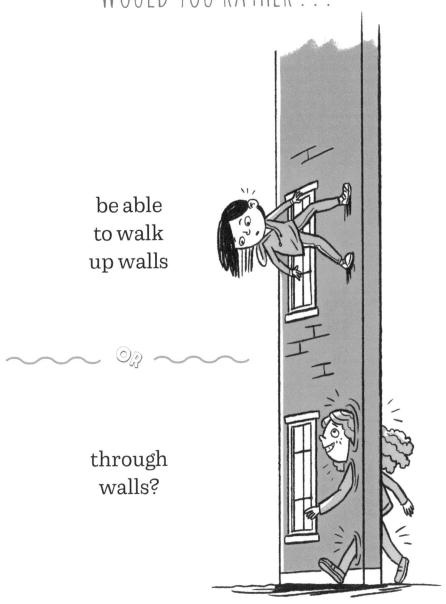

9

IN THE FUTURE

WOULD YOU RATHER . . .

be the first person to discover a new dinosaur species

OR

be the first person to land on Mars?

have to get lots of shots as an adult

OR

have a job where you give people shots?

always drive your car everywhere

OR

have a car that can drive itself so
you can nap in the backseat?

have everything in your house run by a computer,
so you can say, "House, clean my room" or
"House, make me a sandwich" and it happens

OR

have your parents do those things for
you for the rest of your life?

have a family with 10 kids and one cockatiel

OR

one kid and 10 cockatiels?

WOULD YOU RATHER . . .

that people in the future get famous for being rich

OR

for being kind?

get good at skills like playing the piano and making free throw shots through lots and lots of practice

OR

by having the knowledge of how to do these things downloaded instantly into your brain?

we never find aliens living on another planet

OR

we do find aliens and then they turn us all into their pets?

that 30 years from now the number of humans on Earth doubles

OR

the number of animals on Earth doubles?

work eight hours a day for five days a week

OR

ten hours a day for four days a week?

Would you rather . . .

watch basketball played by
remote-controlled robots
OR
video game avatars?

~~~~~~~~~~~~~~~~~~

be a veterinarian when you grow up
OR
a plumber?

~~~~~~~~~~~~~~~~~~

have a computer pick your perfect
life partner for you
OR
try to meet them yourself?

~~~~~~~~~~~~~~~~~~

your future kids go outside to play and explore,
and you don't always know where they are,
OR
they live their entire childhood lives
inside and have all experiences via virtual
reality, so you always know they are safe?

WOULD YOU RATHER . . .

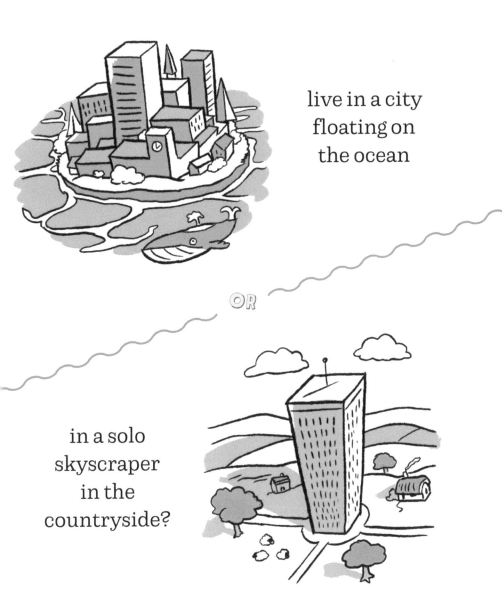

live in a city
floating on
the ocean

OR

in a solo
skyscraper
in the
countryside?

WOULD YOU RATHER . . .

live in a colony on Mars

OR

a spaceship that is traveling across the galaxy?

only take pills for your meals, but the pills taste good,
provide you with the exact right amount of nutrients and
calories you need, and make you feel full

OR

continue eating real food, but sometimes
overeat or not eat enough and not get the
vitamins and minerals you need?

online shop for clothes

OR

3D-print your shiny metallic jumpsuit
so it fits you perfectly?

charge your phone by plugging it into your
solar-energy-gathering shirt

OR

your hat that has a wind turbine on top of it?

Would you rather . . .

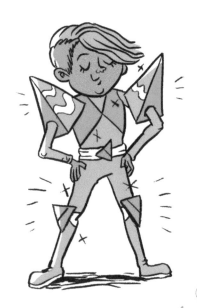

everyone wear shiny metallic jumpsuits with ornate, triangular shoulder pads

OR

jumpsuits that include helmets with antennae sticking out of them?

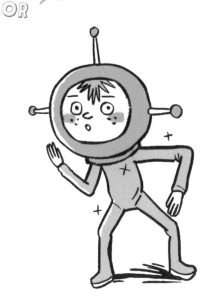

WOULD YOU RATHER . . .

live in a town that regularly experiences earthquakes
OR
tornadoes?

~~~~~~~~~~

have a flying car to get places
OR
a teleportation device that instantly
sends you wherever you need to go?

~~~~~~~~~~

have your mind downloaded into a robot
so you can have a perfect face and body
OR
stick with the body you were born with?

~~~~~~~~~~

live in a tiny, one-room apartment in
a big city with tons of things to do
OR
a huge house in a beautiful place in
the country where cows outnumber people?

~~~~~~~~~~

live right by an amusement park
OR
have your own 50-foot waterslide in your backyard?

WOULD YOU RATHER . . .

become the president of the United States

OR

a gamer with a livestream video feed
that millions of people watch?

have robot pets that will be with you your entire life

OR

real animals as pets, knowing
they won't be around forever?

have windows, pictures, and posters on the walls of
your house

OR

all the walls in your house be giant TV screens,
so you can watch videos everywhere you go?

live in a city where the streets are always full of cars

OR

the sky is always full of drones?

Would you rather . . .

your backyard was a habitat that attracted
all sorts of wild animals you could see from
the windows of your home

OR

it had a swimming pool, a karaoke stage,
and other fun stuff that made it party central
for your friends and family?

that you and everyone else on Earth make
some sacrifices so we can work together to
solve the world's problems before they get worse

OR

you and everyone else do what we want
and enjoy ourselves, and let the next
generations deal with the problems?

have your doctor be a robot

OR

your kids' teacher be a robot?

have your smartphone embedded in your glasses

OR

your brain?

WOULD YOU RATHER . . .

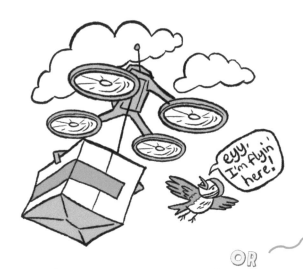

have your packages delivered by robot drones

OR

by delivery people wearing jetpacks?

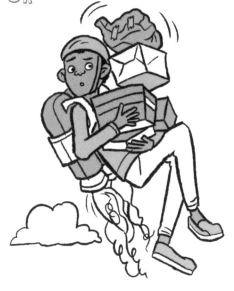

WOULD YOU RATHER . . .

go to a zoo and see live cloned dinosaurs
and mammoths

OR

genetically modified animals, like rabbits
that glow in the dark and mice with
ears growing out of their backs?

eat meat that was grown in a laboratory

OR

eat 3D-printed pizza?

sleep in a tube every night that keeps
your skin from wrinkling

OR

always wear an invisible UV shield around
your body whenever you go outside so you are
protected from the sunlight that causes wrinkling?

become a writer who writes a book of
Would You Rather questions

OR

an artist who draws the illustrations for
a book of Would You Rather questions?

WOULD YOU RATHER . . .

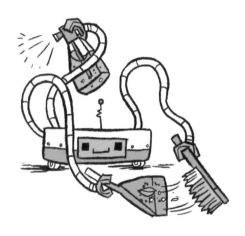

have robots
clean
your house

OR

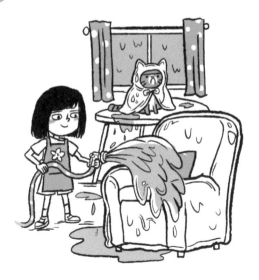

have everything
inside your
house made
of waterproof
plastic you could
hose clean?

10

WRITE YOUR OWN QUESTIONS!

WOULD YOU RATHER . . .

put _____Milk_____ on a hot dog

OR

_____Juice_____?

(fill in two types of condiments or toppings)

wear a ~~~~ Iton Metal helmet on your head

OR

a(n) _Iton pile of cushions_

(fill in two things you can wear or put on your head)

have a(n) _____Dragon_____ as a pet

OR

~~~~ _king kong_?

(fill in two types of animals)

be the best at _Everthing_ at your school

OR

the best at _1 thing_?

(fill in two skills, talents, or school subjects)

become a(n) _____Skydiver_____ when you grow up

OR

a(n) _gymnast_?

(fill in two types of jobs you can have)

WOULD YOU RATHER...

have the magical ability to _Control plants_
OR
Controll lightnig?
(fill in two kinds of superpowers or magical talents)

be the world's best _Javelin thr~~ower~~_
OR
the world's best _speed climb~~er~~_?
(fill in two games or sports)

travel to _Pluto_
OR
each of the stars that make? _up O'rians belt_
(fill in two destinations on Earth or in the universe)

have a huge collection of _games_
OR
a huge collection of _marbles_?
(fill in two types of things that people can collect)

read a book about _a tree_
OR
a book about _a couch_?
(fill in two nonfiction topics or fictional story ideas)

Acknowledgments

Thanks to Sarah Zakalik, Adam Guarnera, Noah Guarnera, and Craig Watkins for giving me some ideas for this book.

About the Author

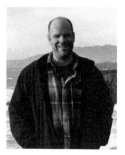

KEVIN KURTZ would rather be a writer than pretty much any other job he can think of. He is an award-winning children's author who specializes in books about science and nature. He also likes that he gets to talk to kids regularly through doing live and virtual school visits. You can learn more about him at KevKurtz.com.

CPSIA information can be obtained
at www.ICGtesting.com
Printed in the USA
JSHW030918241121
20678JS00003B/3